Healthy Keto

Diet

Cookbook

Healthy Keto Diet Recipes For The
Busy Smart People On Keto Diet

Mary Shepard

TABLE OF CONTENTS

INTRODUCTION

The Ketogenic diet is a high-fat, low-carbohydrate diet. It can help reduce your weight by suppressing your appetite, and the keto diet has been shown to improve cholesterol levels, insulin sensitivity and blood sugar control.

The Keto Diet is a restrictive plan because it limits carbs that are natural sugars like breads, cereals, rice and potatoes. It also requires you to cut out fruit because of their natural sugar content. The goal of the Keto Diet is to force your body into a metabolic state called ketosis so that fat stores can be used for energy instead of glucose from carbs or sugar from food which triggers weight loss when you consume less than 10% carbohydrates.

The Ketogenic diet gets its name from the word "ketosis". That is, when your body is almost completely depleted of carbohydrates and glycogen stores, you switch to burning fat for fuel. The end result is a state in which your liver produces small ketone bodies at the same time as your body starts using fat for energy. The process of ketosis takes about 48 hours, but you can encourage it in as little as 24 hours by restricting carbohydrate intake appropriately and fasting.

This low-carb diet forces the body to burn stored fat instead of glucose. With lower insulin levels, stored body fat is released from tissues such as adipose tissue (body fat) and muscles. When the body is forced to burn fat for energy, this is often referred to as "ketosis".

Keto diets have also been linked to a reduced risk of certain diseases such as Type 2 diabetes and Alzheimer's disease. There are many types of keto diets, and the more restrictive ones can be hard to follow, especially if you don't plan ahead. We appreciate that there is a keto diet to suit everyone's food preferences and schedule. We have prepared a short list of the best keto supplements here which can help you get into ketosis quickly and effectively.

The Ketogenic Diet (or Keto Diet) is a low-carb, high-fat diet usually consumed in the form of a fat fast. The purpose of this diet is to force the body into a metabolic state called ketosis. Ketosis occurs when the concentration of ketones in the blood increases and exceeds the amount of carbohydrates. In contrast to a starvation diet, which requires you to eat less than 20 grams of carbohydrates per day, a keto diet doesn't require you to eat as little as 5 percent or less by calories from carbohydrate.

When you're on keto, it helps you lose weight by reducing your appetite so that your body is at reduced risk for overeating. Also, when you're in ketosis, fat and protein intake help keep you feeling full for longer, so you naturally eat less.

This is the foundation of the Keto diet. If you can keep your body in a state of ketosis, which is when your body uses fat as its primary fuel source instead of glucose, you'll experience all sorts of benefits including weight loss.

BREAKFAST

1. Breakfast Meatloaf

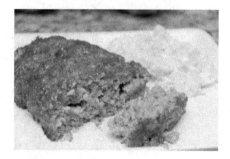

Preparation Time: 18 minutes

Cooking time: 7 hours

Servings: 8

Ingredients:

- 12oz. ground beef
- 1teaspoon salt
- 1teaspoon ground coriander
- 1tablespoon ground mustard
- 1/4teaspoon ground chili pepper
- 6oz. white bread
- 1/2cup milk
- 1teaspoon ground black pepper
- 3tablespoon tomato sauce

Directions:

1. Chop the white bread and combine it with the milk.

2. Stir then set aside for 3 minutes.

3. Meanwhile, combine the ground beef, salt, ground coriander, ground mustard, ground chili pepper, and ground black pepper.

4. Stir the white bread mixture carefully and add it to the ground beef. Cover the slow cooker bowl with foil.

5. Shape the meatloaf and place the uncooked meatloaf in the slow cooker then spread it with the tomato sauce.

6. Close the slow cooker lid and cook

7. Slice the prepared meatloaf and serve. Enjoy!

Nutrition: Calories 214 Fat 14 Carbs 1.2 Protein 9

2. Breakfast Sweet Pepper Rounds

Preparation Time: 10 minutes

Cooking time: 3 hours

Servings: 4

Ingredients

- 2red sweet pepper
- 7oz. ground chicken
- 5oz. Parmesan
- 1tablespoon sour cream
- 1tablespoon flour
- 1egg
- 2teaspoon almond milk
- 1teaspoon salt
- 1/2teaspoon ground black pepper
- 1/4teaspoon butter

Directions:

1. Combine the sour cream with the ground chicken, flour, ground black pepper, almond milk, and butter.
2. Beat eggs into the mixture.
3. Detach the seeds from the sweet peppers and slice them roughly.
4. Place the pepper slices in the slow cooker and fill them with the ground chicken mixture.

5. After this, chop Parmesan into the cubes and add them to the sliced peppers.

6. Close and cook the dish for 3 hours on HIGH.

7. When the time is done make sure that the ground chicken is cooked and the cheese is melted. Enjoy the dish immediately.

Nutrition: Calories 261 Fat 8 Carbs 1.3 Protein 21

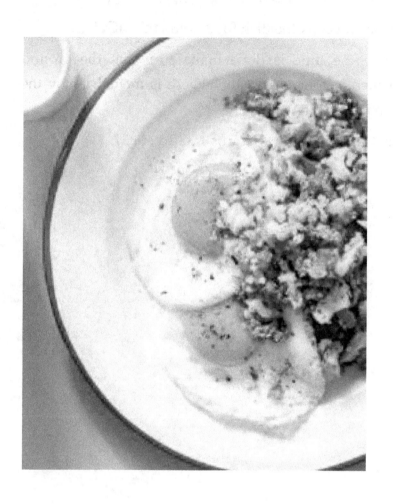

3. Breakfast Cauliflower Hash

Preparation Time: 17 minutes

Cooking time: 8 hours

Servings: 5

Ingredients:

- 7eggs
- 1/4cup milk
- 1teaspoon salt
- 1teaspoon ground black pepper
- 1/2teaspoon ground mustard
- 10oz. cauliflower
- 1/4teaspoon chili flakes
- 5oz. breakfast sausages, chopped
- 1/2onion, chopped
- 5oz. Cheddar cheese, shredded

Directions:

1. Wash the cauliflower carefully and separate it into the florets.
2. After this, shred the cauliflower florets.
3. Beat the eggs and whisk. Add the milk, salt, ground black pepper, ground mustard, chili flakes, and chopped onion into the whisked egg mixture.
4. Put the shredded cauliflower in the slow cooker.

5. Add the whisked egg mixture. Add the shredded cheese and chopped sausages.

6. Stir the mixture gently and close the slow cooker lid.

7. Cook the dish on LOW for 8 hours. When the cauliflower hash is cooked, remove it from the slow cooker and mix up. Enjoy!

Nutrition: Calories 329 Fat 16 Carbs 1.0 Protein 23

4. Savory Creamy Breakfast Casserole

Preparation Time: 17 minutes

Cooking time: 5 hours on low / 3 hours on high

Servings: 5

Ingredients:

- 1tablespoon, extra-virgin olive oil
- 10large eggs, beaten
- 1cup heavy (whipping) cream
- 11/2cups shredded sharp Cheddar cheese, divided
- 1/2cup grated Romano cheese
- 1/2teaspoon kosher salt
- 1/4teaspoon freshly ground black pepper
- 8ounces thick-cut ham, diced
- 3/4 head broccoli, cut into small florets
- 1/2onion, diced

Directions:

1. Brush butter into a cooker.
2. Directly in the insert, whisk together the eggs, heavy cream, 1/2 cup of Cheddar cheese, the Romano cheese, salt, and pepper.
3. Stir in the ham, broccoli, and onion.
4. Cover and cook on low or 3 hours on high. Serve hot.

Nutrition: Calories 465 Fat 10 Carbs 5 Protein 28

5. Bacon & Cheese Frittata

Preparation Time: 15 minutes

Cooking time: 2 hours 30 minutes

Servings: 8

Ingredients:

- 1/2 lb. bacon
- 2tablespoons butter
- 8oz. fresh spinach, packed down
- 10eggs
- 1/2cup heavy whipping cream
- 1/2cup shredded cheese
- Salt and pepper

Directions:

1. Butter or grease the inside of your slow-cooker.
2. Loosely chop the spinach.
3. Cut bacon into half-inch pieces.
4. Beat the eggs with the spices, cream, cheese, and chopped spinach. Then everything will be blended smoothly.
5. Pour the egg mixture over the bacon.
6. Cover the crock pot and adjust the temperature to high
7. Cook for 2 hours. Serve hot.

Nutrition: Calories 392 Fat 34 Carbs 4 Protein 19

LUNCH

6. Carnitas

Preparation time: 15 minutes

Cooking time: 9 hours

Servings: 8

Ingredients:

- 3Tablespoons Extra-Virgin Olive Oil, Divided
- 2Pounds Pork Shoulder, Cut into 2-Inch Cubes
- 2Cups Diced Tomatoes
- 2Cups Chicken Broth
- 1/2Sweet Onion, Chopped
- 2Fresh Chipotle Peppers, Chopped
- Juice of 1 Lime
- 1Teaspoon Ground Coriander
- 1Teaspoon Ground Cumin
- 1/2Teaspoon Salt
- 1Avocado, Peeled, Pitted, And Diced, For Garnish
- 1Cup Sour Cream, For Garnish
- 2Tablespoons Chopped Cilantro, For Garnish

Directions:

1. Lightly grease the insert of the slow cooker with 1 tablespoon of the olive oil.

2. In a large skillet over medium-high heat, heat the remaining 2 tablespoons of the olive oil.

3. Add the pork and brown on all sides for about 10 minutes.

4. Transfer to the insert and add the tomatoes, broth, onion, peppers, lime juice, coriander, cumin, and salt.

5. Cover and cook on low for 9 to 10 hours.

6. Shred the cooked pork with a fork and stir the meat into the sauce.

7. Serve topped with the avocado, sour cream, and cilantro.

Nutrition: Calories 165 Fat 11 g Carbs 5 g Fiber 10 g Sugar 4 g Protein 21 g

7. Asian Pork Spare Ribs

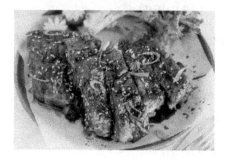

Preparation time: 10 minutes

Cooking time: 9 hours

Servings: 4

Ingredients:

- 1Tablespoon Extra-Virgin Olive Oil
- 2Pounds Pork Spare Ribs
- 1Tablespoon Chinese Five-Spice Powder
- 2Teaspoons Garlic Powder
- 1/2Cup Chicken Broth
- 3Tablespoons Coconut Aminos
- 3Tablespoons Sesame Oil
- 2Tablespoons Apple Cider Vinegar
- 1Tablespoon Granulated Erythritol

Directions:

1. Lightly grease the insert of the slow cooker with the olive oil.

2. Season the ribs with the five-spice powder and garlic powder, and place upright on their ends in the insert.

3. Add the broth, coconut aminos, sesame oil, apple cider vinegar, and erythritol to the bottom of the insert, stirring to blend.

4. Cover and cook on low for 9 to 10 hours.

5. Serve warm.

Nutrition: Calories 176 Fat 9 g Carbs 4 g Fiber 9 g Sugar 3 g Protein 27 g

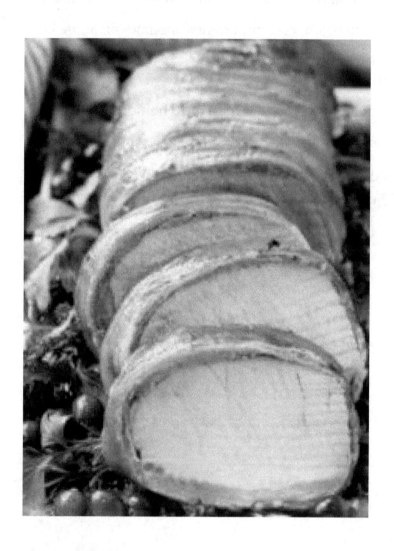

8. Bacon-Wrapped Pork Loin

Preparation time: 15 minutes

Cooking time: 9 hours

Servings: 6

Ingredients:

- 3Tablespoons Extra-Virgin Olive Oil, Divided
- 2Pounds Pork Shoulder Roast
- 1Teaspoon Garlic Powder
- 1Teaspoon Onion Powder
- 8Bacon Strips, Uncooked
- 1/4Cup Chicken Broth
- 2Teaspoons Chopped Thyme
- 1Teaspoon Chopped Oregano

Directions:

1. Lightly grease the insert of the slow cooker with 1 tablespoon of the olive oil.

2. Rub the pork all over with the garlic powder and onion powder.

3. In a large skillet over medium-high heat, heat the remaining 2 tablespoons of the olive oil. Add the pork to the skillet and brown on all sides for about 10 minutes. Let stand about 10 minutes to cool.

4. Wrap the pork with the bacon slices, place in the insert, and add the broth, thyme, and oregano.

5. Cover and cook on low for 9 to 10 hours.

6. Serve warm.

Nutrition: Calories 312 Fat 8 g Carbs 3 g Fiber 12 g Sugar 8 g Protein 25 g

9. All-In-One Lamb-Vegetable Dinner

Preparation time: 10 minutes

Cooking time: 6 hours

Servings: 4

Ingredients:

- 1/4Cup Extra-Virgin Olive Oil, Divided
- 1Pound Boneless Lamb Chops, About 1/2-Inch Thick
- Salt, For Seasoning
- Freshly Ground Black Pepper, For Seasoning
- 1/2Sweet Onion, Sliced
- 1/2Fennel Bulb., Cut into 2-Inch Chunks
- 1Zucchini, Cut into 1-Inch Chunks
- 1/4Cup Chicken Broth
- 2Tablespoons Chopped Fresh Basil, For Garnish

Directions:

1. Lightly grease the insert of the slow cooker with 1 tablespoon of the olive oil.

2. Season the lamb with salt and pepper.

3. In a medium bowl, toss together the onion, fennel, and zucchini with the remaining 3 tablespoons of the olive oil and then place half of the vegetables in the insert.

4. Place the lamb on top of the vegetables, cover with the remaining vegetables, and add the broth.

5. Cover and cook on low for 6 hours.

6. Serve topped with the basil.

Nutrition: Calories 254 Fat 8 g Carbs 3 g Fiber 12 g Sugar 8 g Protein 27 g

10. Wild Mushroom Lamb Shanks

Preparation time: 15 minutes

Cooking time: 7 hours

Servings: 6

Ingredients:

- 3Tablespoons Extra-Virgin Olive Oil, Divided
- 2Pounds Lamb Shanks
- 1/2Pound Wild Mushrooms, Sliced
- 1Leek, Thoroughly Cleaned and Chopped
- 2Celery Stalks, Chopped
- 1Carrot, Diced
- 1Tablespoon Minced Garlic
- 1Can Crushed Tomatoes
- 1/2Cup Beef Broth
- 2Tablespoons Apple Cider Vinegar
- 1Teaspoon Dried Rosemary
- 1/2 Cup Sour Cream, For Garnish

Directions:

1. Lightly grease the insert of the slow cooker with 1 tablespoon of the olive oil.

2. In a large skillet over medium-high heat, heat the remaining 2 tablespoons of the olive oil. Add the lamb;

brown for 6 minutes, turning once; and transfer to the insert.

3. In the skillet, sauté the mushrooms, leek, celery, carrot, and garlic for 5 minutes.

4. Transfer the vegetables to the insert along with the tomatoes, broth, apple cider vinegar, and rosemary.

5. Cover and cook on low for 7 to 8 hours.

6. Serve topped with the sour cream.

Nutrition: Calories 187 Fat 12 g Carbs 2.9 g Fiber 9 g Sugar 3 g Protein 21 g

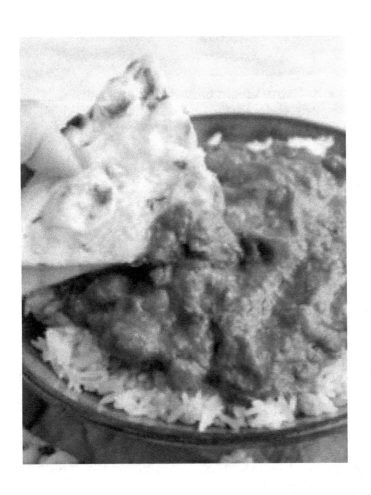

11. Curried Lamb

Preparation time: 15 minutes

Cooking time: 7 hours

Servings: 6

Ingredients:

- 3Tablespoons Extra-Virgin Olive Oil, Divided
- 11/2Pounds Lamb Shoulder Chops
- Salt, For Seasoning
- Freshly Ground Black Pepper, For Seasoning
- 3Cups Coconut Milk
- 1/2Sweet Onion, Sliced
- 1/4Cup Curry Powder
- 1Tablespoon Grated Fresh Ginger
- 2Teaspoons Minced Garlic
- 1Carrot, Diced
- 2Tablespoons Chopped Cilantro, For Garnish

Directions:

1. Lightly grease the insert of the slow cooker with 1 tablespoon of the olive oil.

2. In a large skillet over medium-high heat, heat the remaining 2 tablespoons of the olive oil.

3. Season the lamb with salt and pepper. Add the lamb to the skillet and brown for 6 minutes, turning once. Transfer to the insert.

4. In a medium bowl, stir together the coconut milk, onion, curry, ginger, and garlic.

5. Add the mixture to the lamb along with the carrot.

6. Cover and cook on low for 7 to 8 hours.

7. Serve topped with the cilantro.

Nutrition: Calories 287 Fat 21 g Carbs 5 g Fiber 11 g Sugar 5 g Protein 12 g

12. Rosemary Lamb Chops

Preparation time: 15 minutes

Cooking time: 6 hours

Servings: 4

Ingredients:

- 3Tablespoons Extra-Virgin Olive Oil, Divided
- 11/2Pounds Lamb Shoulder Chops
- Salt, For Seasoning
- Freshly Ground Black Pepper, For Seasoning
- 1/2Cup Chicken Broth
- 1Sweet Onion, Sliced
- 2Teaspoons Minced Garlic
- 2Teaspoons Dried Rosemary
- 1Teaspoon Dried Thyme

Directions:

1. Lightly grease the insert of the slow cooker with 1 tablespoon of the olive oil.

2. In a large skillet over medium-high heat, heat the remaining 2 tablespoons of the olive oil.

3. Season the lamb with salt and pepper. Add the lamb to the skillet and brown for 6 minutes, turning once.

4. Transfer the lamb to the insert, and add the broth, onion, garlic, rosemary, and thyme.

5. Cover and cook on low for 6 hours.

6. Serve warm.

Nutrition: Calories 145 Fat 21 g Carbs 3 g Fiber 13 g Sugar 5 g Protein 18 g

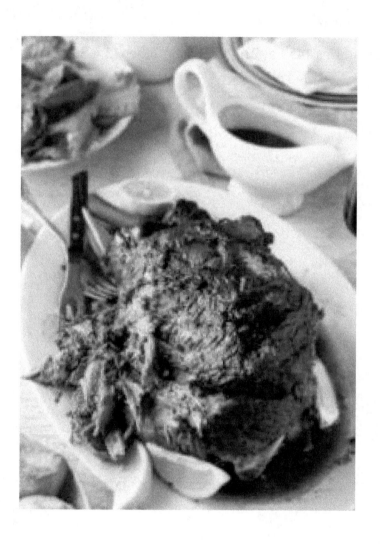

13. Tender Lamb Roast

Preparation time: 10 minutes

Cooking time: 8 hours

Servings: 6

Ingredients:

- 1Tablespoon Extra-Virgin Olive Oil
- 2Pounds Lamb Shoulder Roast
- Salt, For Seasoning
- Freshly Ground Black Pepper, For Seasoning
- 1Can Diced Tomatoes
- 1Tablespoon Cumin
- 2Teaspoons Minced Garlic
- 1Teaspoon Paprika
- 1Teaspoon Chili Powder
- 1Cup Sour Cream
- 2Teaspoons Chopped Fresh Parsley, For Garnish

Directions:

1. Lightly grease the insert of the slow cooker with the olive oil.
2. Lightly season the lamb with salt and pepper.
3. Place the lamb in the insert and add the tomatoes, cumin, garlic, paprika, and chili powder.
4. Cover and cook on low for 7 to 8 hours.

5. Stir in the sour cream.

6. Serve topped with the parsley.

Nutrition: Calories 391 Fat 12 g Carbs 2 g Fiber 11 g Sugar 5 g Protein 28 g

14. Flavorful Mexican Cheese Dip

Preparation time: 10 minutes

Cooking time: 1hours

Servings: 6

Ingredients:

- 1tsp. taco seasoning
- 1oz. Velveeta cheese, cut into cube
- 3/4cup tomatoes with green chilies

Directions:

1. Add cheese into the slow cooker. Cover and cook on low for 30 minutes. Stir occasionally.
2. Add taco seasoning and tomatoes with green chilies and stir well.
3. Cover again and cook on low for 30 minutes more.
4. Stir well and serve.

Nutrition: Calories 243 Fat 21 g Carbs 2.1 g Fiber 13 g Sugar 1 g Protein 21 g

15. Salsa Beef Dip

Preparation time: 10 minutes

Cooking time: 1 hour

Servings: 20

Ingredients:

- 32Oz. salsa
- 1lb. ground beef
- 1lb. Velveeta cheese, cubed

Directions:

1. Brown beef in a pan over medium heat. Drain well and transfer to the slow cooker. Add cheese and salsa and stir well.

2. Cover slow cooker with lid and cook on high for 1 hour.

3. Stir well and serve.

Nutrition: Calories 165 Fat 12 g Carbs 2.1 g Fiber 11 g Sugar 4 g Protein 24 g

DINNER

16. Cod & Peas with Sour Cream

Preparation Time: 6 minutes

Cooking time: 1 hr.

Servings: 6

Ingredients

- 1 tablespoon of fresh parsley
- 1 garlic clove, diced
- 1/2 lb. frozen peas
- 1/2 teaspoon of paprika
- 1 cup of sour cream
- 1/2 cup of white wine

Directions:

1. Start by throwing all the Ingredients: into your Crockpot except sour cream.
2. Cover its lid and cook for 1 hour on High setting.
3. Once done, remove its lid and give it a stir.
4. Stir in sour cream and mix it gently
5. Serve warm.

Nutrition: Calories 349 Fat 31.9 g Sodium 237 mg Carbs 1.6 g Sugar 1.4 g Fiber 3.4 g Protein 11 g

17. Slow Cooker Tuna Steaks

Preparation Time: 6 minutes

Cooking time: 4 hrs.

Servings: 6

Ingredients

- 4 tuna steaks
- 3 garlic cloves, crushed
- 1 lemon, sliced into 8 slices
- 1/2 cup white wine

Directions:

1. Reduce the white wine in a pot by simmering until the strong alcoholic smell is cooked off.
2. Rub the tuna steaks with olive oil, and sprinkle with salt and pepper.
3. Place the tuna steaks into the Slow Cooker.
4. Sprinkle the crushed garlic on top of the tuna steaks.
5. Place 2 lemon slices on top of each tuna steak.
6. Pour the reduced wine into the pot.
7. Secure the lid onto the pot and set the temperature to HIGH.
8. Cook for 3 hours.
9. Serve with a drizzle of leftover liquid from the pot, and a side of crispy greens!

Nutrition: Calories 123 Fat 21 g Sodium 213 mg Carbs 2 g Sugar 2 g Fiber 3g Protein 15 g

18. Tilapia and Radish Bites

Preparation Time: 5 minutes

Cooking time: 2 hrs.

Servings: 2

Ingredients

- 1 1/2 cups radishes, halved
- 1 teaspoon sweet paprika
- 1/2 teaspoon dried rosemary
- 1/4 teaspoon ground black pepper
- 1/2 teaspoon salt
- 9 oz. tilapia fillet, boneless and cubed
- 2 oz. Cheddar cheese, sliced
- 1/4 cup veggie stock

Directions:

1. In the slow cooker, mix the radishes with the fish and the other ingredients and toss.
2. Close the lid and cook the fish for 5 hours on High.

Nutrition: Calories 251, Fat 8.4, Fiber 0.2, Carbs 1.3, Protein 6.6

19. Shrimp & Pepper Stew

Preparation Time: 5 minutes

Cooking time: 2 hrs.

Servings: 4

Ingredients

- 14 oz. canned diced tomatoes
- 1/4 cup of yellow onion, peeled and diced
- 2 tablespoon of lime juice
- 1/4 cup of olive oil
- 11/2 lbs. shrimp, peeled and deveined
- 1/4 cup of red pepper, roasted and diced
- 1 garlic clove, peeled and diced
- 1 cup of coconut milk
- 1/4 cup of fresh cilantro, diced
- Salt and black pepper ground, to taste

Directions:

1. Start by throwing all the Ingredients: into your Crockpot except shrimp.
2. Cover its lid and cook for 2 hours on Low setting.
3. Once done, remove its lid and give it a stir.
4. Stir in shrimp and continue cooking for 1 hour on low heat.
5. Serve warm.

Nutrition: Calories 392 Fat 40.4 g Sodium 423 mg Carbs 2.7 g Sugar 3 g Protein 21 g

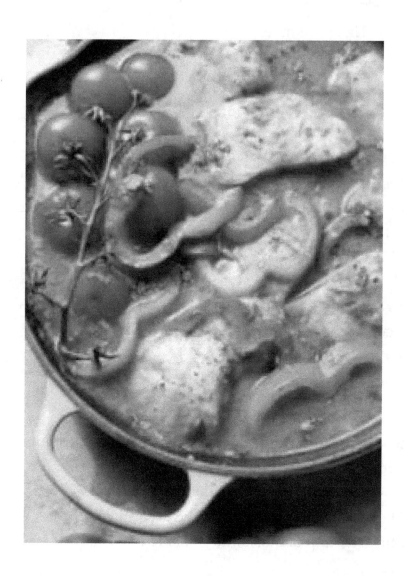

20. Seafood Stew

Preparation Time: 5 minutes

Cooking time: 4 hrs.

Servings: 4

Ingredients

- Haddock fillets – 1/2 lb., cut into 1-inch pieces
- Raw shrimp – 1/2 lb., peeled, deveined
- Lump crab meat – 1/2 (6 oz.) can, drained
- Chopped clams – 1/2 (6 oz.) can, with its liquid
- Clam juice – 4 oz.
- Olive oil – 1/2 tbsp.
- Medium onion – 1, chopped
- Garlic – 3 cloves, minced
- Celery – 2 ribs, chopped
- Tomato paste – 1/2 (6 oz.) can
- Diced tomatoes – 1/2 (28 oz.) can, with liquid
- White wine – 1/4 cup
- Red wine vinegar – 1/2 tbsp.
- Italian seasoning – 1 tsp.
- Bay leaf – 1
- Erythritol – 1/4 tsp.
- Parsley – 2 tbsp. chopped
- Salt to taste

Directions:

1. Except for seafood and parsley, add all the ingredients to the Crock-Pot.
2. Cover and cook on low for 3 to 4 hours.

3. Add the seafood and mix well.
4. Cover and cook on high for 30 minutes. Stir a couple of times while it is cooking.
5. Discard the bay leaf. Add parsley.
6. Mix well and serve.

Nutrition: Calories: 201 Fat: 4g Carbs: 1.8g Protein: 30.4g

21. Creamy Seafood Chowder

Preparation Time: 5 minutes

Cooking time: 5 hrs.

Servings: 6

Ingredients

- Garlic – 5 cloves, crushed
- Small onion – 1, finely chopped
- Prawns – 1 cup
- Shrimp – 1 cup
- Whitefish – 1 cup
- Full-fat cream – 2 cups
- Dry white wine – 1 cup
- A handful of fresh parsley, finely chopped
- Olive oil – 2 tbsp.

Directions:

1. Drizzle oil into the Crock-Pot.
2. Add the white fish, shrimp, prawns, onion, garlic, cream, wine, salt, and pepper into the pot. Stir to mix.
3. Cover with the lid and cook on low for 5 hours.
4. Sprinkle with fresh parsley and serve.

Nutrition: Calories: 225 Fat: 9.6g Carbs: 5.g Protein: 21.4g

22. <u>Salmon Cake</u>

Preparation Time: 5 minutes

Cooking time: 4 hrs.

Servings: 4

Ingredients

- Eggs – 4, lightly beaten
- Heavy cream – 3 tbsp.
- Baby spinach – 1 cup, roughly chopped
- Smoked salmon strips – 4 ounces, chopped
- A handful of fresh coriander, roughly chopped
- Olive oil – 2 tbsp.
- Salt and pepper to taste

Directions:

1. Drizzle oil into the Crock-Pot.
2. Place the spinach, cream, beaten egg, salmon, salt, and pepper into the pot and mix to combine.
3. Cover with the lid and cook on low for 4 hours.
4. Sprinkle with fresh coriander and serve.

Nutrition: Calories: 277 Fat: 20.8g Carbs: 1.1g Protein: 22.5g

23. Lemon-Butter Fish

Preparation Time: 5 minutes

Cooking time: 5 hrs.

Servings: 4

Ingredients

- Fresh white fish – 4 fillets
- Butter - 1 1/2 ounce, soft but not melted
- Garlic cloves – 2, crushed
- Lemon – 1 (juice and zest)
- A handful of fresh parsley, finely chopped
- Salt and pepper to taste
- Olive oil – 2 tbsp.

Directions:

1. Combine the butter, garlic, zest of one lemon, and chopped parsley to a bowl.
2. Drizzle oil into the Crock-Pot.
3. Season the fish with salt and pepper and place into the pot.
4. Place a dollop of lemon butter onto each fish fillet and gently spread it out.
5. Cover with the lid and cook on low for 5 hours.
6. Serve each fish fillet with a generous spoonful of melted lemon butter from the bottom of the pot. Drizzle with lemon juice and serve.

Nutrition: Calories: 202 Fat: 13.4g Carbs: 1.3g Protein: 20.3g

24. Salmon with Green Beans

Preparation Time: 5 minutes

Cooking time: 3 hrs.

Servings: 4

Ingredients

- Salmon fillets – 4, skin on
- Garlic – 4 cloves, crushed
- Broccoli – 1/2 head, cut into florets
- Frozen green beans – 2 cups
- Olive oil – 3 tbsp., divided
- Salt and pepper to taste
- Water – 1/4 cup

Directions:

1. Add the olive oil into the Crock-Pot.
2. Season the salmon with salt and pepper and place into the pot (skin-side down). Add the water.
3. Place garlic, beans, and broccoli on top of the salmon. Season with salt and pepper.
4. Drizzle some more oil over the veggies and fish.
5. Cover with the lid and cook on high for 3 hours.
6. Serve.

Nutrition: Calories: 278 Fat: 17.8g Carbs: 1g Protein: 24.5g

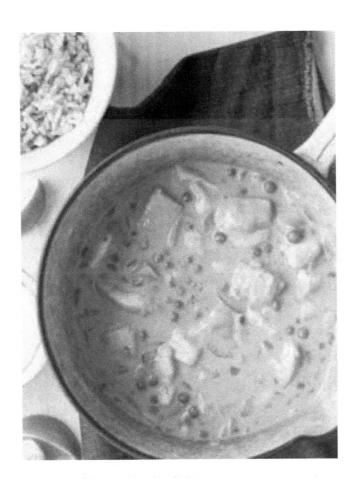

25. Coconut Fish Curry

Preparation Time: 5 minutes

Cooking time: 4 hrs.

Servings: 4

Ingredients

- Large white fish fillets – 4, cut into chunks
- Garlic cloves – 4, crushed
- Small onion – 1, finely chopped
- Ground turmeric – 1 tsp.
- Yellow curry paste – 2 tbsp.
- Fish stock – 2 cups
- Full-fat coconut milk – 2 cans
- Lime – 1
- Fresh coriander as needed, roughly chopped
- Olive oil – 2 tbsp.
- Salt and pepper to taste

Directions:

1. Add olive oil into the Crock-Pot.

2. Add the coconut milk, stock, fish, curry paste, turmeric, onion, garlic, salt, and pepper to the pot. Stir to combine.

3. Cover with the lid and cook on high for 4 hours.

4. Drizzle with lime juice and fresh coriander and serve.

Nutrition: Calories: 562 Fat: 49.9g Carbs: 1.3g Protein: 20.6g

26. Coconut Lime Mussels

Preparation Time: 5 minutes

Cooking time: 2 hrs.

Servings: 4

Ingredients

- Fresh mussels – 16
- Garlic – 4 cloves
- Full-fat coconut milk – 1 1/2 cups
- Red chili – 1/2, finely chopped
- Lime – 1, juiced
- Fish stock – 1/2 cup
- A handful of fresh coriander
- Olive oil – 2 tbsp.
- Salt and pepper to taste

Directions:

1. Add olive oil into the Crock-Pot.
2. Add the coconut milk, garlic, chili, fish stock, salt, pepper, and juice of one lime to the pot. Stir to mix.
3. Cover with the lid and cook on high for 2 hours.
4. Remove the lid, place mussels into the liquid, and cover with the lid.
5. Cook until mussels open, about 20 minutes.
6. Serve the mussels with pot sauce. Garnish with fresh coriander.

Nutrition: Calories: 342 Fat: 30.2g Carbs: 1.3g Protein: 10.9g

27. Calamari, Prawn, and Shrimp Pasta Sauce

Preparation Time: 5 minutes

Cooking time: 3 hrs.

Servings: 6

Ingredients

- Calamari – 1 cup
- Prawns – 1 cup
- Shrimp – 1 cup
- Garlic – 6 cloves, crushed
- Tomatoes – 4, chopped
- Dried mixed herbs – 1 tsp.
- Balsamic vinegar - 1 tbsp.
- Olive oil – 2 tbsp.
- Salt and pepper to taste
- Water – 1/2 cup

Directions:

1. Add oil into the Crock-Pot.
2. Add the tomatoes, garlic, shrimp, prawns, calamari, mixed herbs, balsamic vinegar, water, salt, and pepper. Stir to mix.
3. Cover with the lid and cook on high for 3 hours.
4. Serve with zucchini noodles or veggies.

Nutrition: Calories: 372 Fat: 14.6g Carbs: 5g Protein: 55.1g

28. Sesame Prawns

Preparation Time: 5 minutes

Cooking time: 2 hrs.

Servings: 4

Ingredients

- Large prawns – 3 cups
- Garlic – 4 cloves, crushed
- Sesame oil – 1 tbsp.
- Toasted sesame seeds – 2 tbsp.
- Red chili – 1/2, finely chopped
- Fish stock – 1/2 cup
- Salt and pepper to taste
- Chopped herbs for serving

Directions:

1. Drizzle the sesame oil into the Crock-Pot.
2. Add the garlic, prawns, sesame seeds, chili, and fish stock to the pot. Mix to coat.
3. Cover with the lid and cook on high for 2 hours.
4. Serve hot with fresh herbs and cauliflower rice.

Nutrition: Calories: 236 Fat: 7.7g Carbs: 4.3g Protein: 37.4g

29. **Tuna Steaks**

Preparation Time: 5 minutes

Cooking time: 3 hrs.

Servings: 4

Ingredients

- Tuna steaks – 4
- Garlic – 3 cloves, crushed
- Lemon – 1, sliced into 8 slices
- White wine – 1/2 cup
- Olive oil – 2 tbsp.
- Salt and pepper to taste

Directions:

1. Reduce the white wine in a pan by simmering until the strong alcohol smell is cooked off.
2. Rub the tuna steaks with olive oil, and season with salt and pepper.
3. Place the tuna steaks into the Crock-Pot.
4. Sprinkle the crushed garlic on top of the tuna steaks.
5. Place 2 lemon slices on top of each tuna steak.
6. Pour the reduced wine into the pot.
7. Cover with the lid and cook on high for 3 hours.
8. Transfer fish on serving plates. Drizzle with pot liquid and serve.

Nutrition: Calories: 269 Fat: 8.6g Carbs: 2.9g Protein: 40.4g

30. Cheese and Prawns

Preparation Time: 5 minutes

Cooking time: 1 hr.

Servings: 4

Ingredients

- Shallots – 2, finely chopped
- Apple cider vinegar – 1/4 cup
- Butter – 2 tbsp.
- Raw prawns – 4 lbs., peeled, rinsed, patted dry
- Almond meal – 2 tsp.
- Swiss cheese – 1 cup, grated
- Garlic – 2 cloves, peeled, thinly sliced
- Hot pepper sauce – 1/4 tsp.
- Salt to taste
- Fresh parsley to serve

Directions:

1. Melt butter in a skillet over medium heat. Then add shallots and sauté for a few minutes until translucent.
2. Add prawns and sauté for 2 minutes. Set aside.
3. Grease the inside of the pot with a little butter.
4. Sprinkle garlic over it and add cheese.
5. In a bowl, mix almond meal, apple cider, and hot sauce. Pour the mixture into the Crock-Pot. Stir.
6. Cover and cook on low for 1 hour.
7. Add the prawn shallot mixture and stir.
8. Cover and cook on low for 10 minutes.
9. Stir again and sprinkle parsley over it.

10. Serve.

Nutrition: Calories: 238 Fat: 13.5g Carbs: 4g Protein: 20g

SNACKS RECIPES

31. Corn Coconut Pudding

Preparation Time: 5 Minutes

Cooking Time: 45 minutes

Servings: 3

Ingredients:

- 3cups water
- 1cup corn kernels
- 1/2cup sticky rice
- 1/4cup ripe jackfruit, shredded,
- 1/4tsp. vanilla extract
- 1/2cup sugar
- 1/8tsp. nutmeg powder
- 1/16tsp. salt
- 2cans thick coconut cream, divided

Directions:

1. Pour water, sticky rice, jackfruit, corn kernels, 1 can of coconut cream, nutmeg powder, vanilla extract, white sugar, and salt in the Instant Pot Pressure Cooker.

2. Lock the lid in place. Press the high pressure and cook for 7 minutes.

3. When the beep sounds, Choose the Quick Pressure Release. This will depressurize for 7 minutes. Remove the lid.

4. Tip in the remaining can of coconut cream. Allow residual heat cook the coconut cream. Adjust seasoning according to your preferred taste.

5. To serve, ladle equal amounts into dessert bowls.

Nutrition: Calories 213 Fat 12 Fiber 21 Carbs 2 Protein 13

32. Raspberry Chocolate Parfait

Preparation Time: 5 Minutes

Cooking Time: 45 minutes

Servings: 3

Ingredients:

- Raspberry chia seeds
- 3Tbsp. chia seeds
- 1cup frozen raspberries, reserve some for garnish
- 1/8tsp. lemon juice, freshly squeezed
- 1/2cup unsweetened almond milk
- 1/4tsp. sugar
- 1/8cup seed tapioca
- 1/2Tbsp. cocoa powder
- 1bar dark chocolate, chopped, reserve some for garnish
- 1cup unsweetened almond milk
- 1cup water

Directions:

1. For the raspberry chia seeds, combine chia seeds, raspberries, almond milk, lemon juice, and white sugar. Mash berries. Mix ingredients well. Cover with saran wrap and place inside the fridge for 1 hour or until ready to use.

2. To make chocolate tapioca, combine dark chocolate, tapioca, cocoa powder, almond milk, and water.

3. Lock the lid in place. Press the high pressure and cook for 10 minutes.

4. When the beep sounds, Choose Natural Pressure Release. Depressurizing would take 20 minutes. Remove the lid.

5. To serve, spoon just the right amount of chocolate tapioca in glasses. Top with raspberry-chia mixture. Garnish with chopped chocolate and fresh raspberries.

Nutrition: Calories 213 Fat 12 Fiber 21 Carbs 2 Protein 13

33. Berry Jam with Chia Seeds

Preparation Time: 5 Minutes

Cooking Time: 45 minutes

Servings: 3

Ingredients:

- 2cups fresh blueberries, stemmed
- 11/2cups water
- 1cup fresh raspberries, stemmed
- 1cup sugar
- 1/16tsp. salt
- 1/2cup chia seeds
- 1/4Tbsp. lemon juice, freshly squeezed

Directions

1. Place raspberries, blueberries, water, sugar, and salt into the Instant Pot Pressure Cooker. Stir.

2. Lock the lid in place. Press the high pressure and cook for 3 minutes.

3. When the beep sounds, Choose the Quick Pressure Release. This will depressurize for 7 minutes. Remove the lid.

4. Add in chia seeds and lemon juice.

5. Process jam into desired consistency using a potato masher. You may choose to have your jam smooth or

chunky. Allow to cool before storing jam into an airtight container. Use as needed.

Nutrition: Calories 128 Fat 11 Fiber 13 Carbs 4.8 Protein 12

34. Apple Risotto

Preparation Time: 5 Minutes

Cooking Time: 45 minutes

Servings: 3

Ingredients:

- 1/2cup apples, sliced into thick disks
- 11/2cups barley pearls
- 1/4tsp. cinnamon powder
- 2cups water
- 1cup apple juice
- 1cup cashew milk
- 1/4cup cashew nuts, chopped
- 1/8tsp. nutmeg powder
- 1/4cup sugar

Directions:

1. Place apples, apple juice, barley pearls, water, cinnamon powder, cashew nuts, cashew milk, nutmeg powder, and sugar inside the Instant Pot Pressure Cooker.

2. Lock the lid in place. Press the high pressure and cook for 7 minutes.

3. When the beep sounds, Choose the Quick Pressure Release. This will depressurize for 7 minutes. Remove

the lid. Adjust seasoning according to your preferred taste.

4. To serve, ladle equal amounts into dessert bowls.

Nutrition: Calories 128 Fat 11 Fiber 13 Carbs 4.8 Protein 12

35. **Nectarines with Dried Cloves**

Preparation Time: 5 Minutes

Cooking Time: 50 minutes

Servings: 4

Ingredients:

- 4dried cloves, whole
- 2lb.s. nectarine, cubed
- 1/4cup agave sugar, reserve for garnish
- 1/16tsp. cinnamon powder
- 2cups water

Directions:

1. Combine dried cloves, nectarine, water, cinnamon powder, and agave sugar into the Instant Pot Pressure Cooker.
2. Lock the lid in place. Press the high pressure and cook for 5 minutes.
3. When the beep sounds, Choose the Quick Pressure Release. This will depressurize for 7 minutes. Remove the lid. Discard dried cloves.
4. To serve, ladle just the right amount into dessert bowls. Sprinkle agave sugar.

Nutrition: Calories 267 Fat 23 Fiber 19 Carbs 5 Protein 21

36. **Chocolate Raspberry Parfait**

Preparation Time: 5 Minutes

Cooking Time: 50 minutes

Servings: 2

Ingredients:

- Raspberry chia seeds
- 3Tbsp. chia seeds
- 1/2cup almond milk, unsweetened
- 1/4tsp. sugar
- 1cup frozen raspberries, reserve some for garnish
- 1/8tsp. lemon juice, freshly squeezed
- Chocolate tapioca
- 1/2Tbsp. Dutch cocoa powder
- 1/8cup seed tapioca, picked over
- 1cup almond milk, unsweetened
- 1cup water
- 4 squares dark chocolate, chopped, reserve some for garnish

Directions

1. For the raspberry chia seeds, combine chia seeds, almond milk, sugar, raspberries, and lemon juice in a bowl. Mix well. Mash berries. Seal with saran wrap. Place inside the fridge until ready to use.

2. For the chocolate tapioca, put together cocoa powder, tapioca, almond milk, water, and dark chocolate into the crockpot. Stir.

3. Lock the lid in place. Press the high pressure and cook for 8 minutes.

4. When the beep sounds, Choose Natural Pressure Release. Depressurizing would take 20 minutes. Remove the lid.

5. To serve, spoon in half portions of chocolate tapioca in heat-proof glass. Put just the right amount of raspberry-chia mixture on top. Garnish with whole raspberries and chopped chocolate.

Nutrition: Calories 321 Fat 22 Fiber 11 Carbs 4 Protein 26

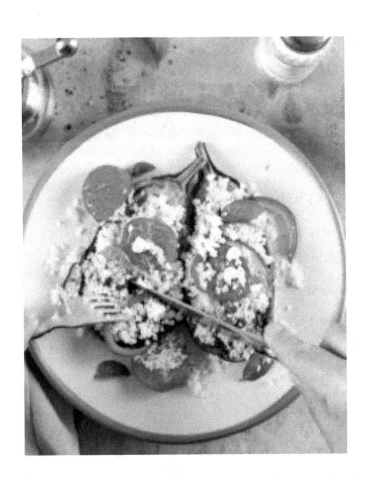

37. **Partings In Moderation**

Preparation Time: 5 Minutes

Cooking Time: 55 minutes

Servings: 6

Ingredients:

- 1/4cup dried red kidney beans, picked over
- 1cup dried Adzuki beans, picked over
- 1/4cup dried pinto beans, picked over
- 6cups water
- 1/2Tbsp. coconut oil
- 1cup brown sugar
- 1/16tsp. green tea powder
- 1/2cup loosely packed shaved ice, per person, prepare this only when about to serve
- 1/4cup almond milk, chilled

Directions:

1. For the bean base, place red kidney beans, adzuki beans, pinto beans, water, and coconut oil into the Instant Pot Pressure Cooker. Stir well.

2. Lock the lid in place. Press the high pressure and cook for 30 minutes.

3. When the beep sounds, Choose Natural Pressure Release. Depressurizing would take 20 minutes. Remove the lid.

4. Drain beans and reserve at least half of the cooking liquid. Put back into the crockpot.

5. Press the "Sauté" button. Stir in brown sugar. Turn off the machine immediately. Let it for 15 minutes or until it thickens.

6. To serve, place shaved ice into bowls. Spoon just the right amount of bean base. Garnish with green tea powder. Drizzle in almond milk. Serve.

Nutrition: Calories 216 Fat 32 Fiber 11 Carbs 4.9 Protein 26

38. Coconut Brown Rice Cake

Preparation Time: 5 Minutes

Cooking Time: 55 minutes

Servings: 6

Ingredients:

- 1cup brown rice
- 1/2cup coconut flakes, for garnish
- 1/4cup raisins
- 2cans thick coconut cream, reserve 3 tsp. for garnish
- 1/8tsp. coconut oil, for greasing
- 1/2cup water
- 1/4cup brown sugar

Directions:

1. Pour coconut flakes into the Instant Pot Pressure Cooker. Press the "sauté" button. Toast flakes until lightly brown. Set aside.

2. Meanwhile, lightly grease the sides and bottom of the pressure cooker.

3. Add in brown rice, 1 can coconut cream, water brown sugar, and raisins.

4. Lock the lid in place. Press the high pressure and cook for 30 minutes.

5. When the beep sounds, Choose Natural Pressure Release. Depressurizing would take 20 minutes. Remove the lid.

6. To serve, place just the right amount of rice cake in a dessert plate. Put coconut flakes on top. Spoon coconut cream.

Nutrition: Calories 216 Fat 32 Fiber 11 Carbs 4.9 Protein 26

39. Rice Dumplings in Coconut Sauce

Preparation Time: 5 Minutes

Cooking Time: 45 minutes

Servings: 4

Ingredients:

- 1/2cup glutinous rice flour
- 1/4cup water
- 2Tbsp. heaping tapioca pearls, uncooked, picked over
- 2cans 15 oz. each thick coconut cream, divided
- 1/4cup sugar
- 1/16tsp. salt
- 2cups water
- 1/2 cup fresh ripe jackfruits, shredded, reserved half for garnish

Directions:

1. For the dumplings, put together glutinous rice flour and water in a bowl. Massage until dough forms into a soft ball. Seal bowl with saran wrap. Let the dough rest for 5 minutes.

2. Roll dough in the palm of your hands. Place on a baking sheet lined with parchment paper. Repeat the same procedure for the rest of the dumplings. Set aside.

3. For the coconut sauce, pour tapioca pearls, 1 can of coconut cream, sugar, salt, water, and ripe jackfruit into the Instant Pot Pressure Cooker

4. Lock the lid in place. Press the high pressure and cook for 7 minutes.

5. When the beep sounds, Choose the Quick Pressure Release. This will depressurize for 7 minutes. Remove the lid.

6. Press the "Sauté" button once again. Bring coconut sauce to a boil.

7. Drop dumplings or until they rise to the top of the cooking liquid. Do not stir.

8. Turn off the machine. Stir in remaining can of coconut cream. Adjust seasoning according to your preferred taste.

9. To serve, ladle equal amounts into dessert bowls. Garnish with shredded jackfruits.

Nutrition: Calories 149 Fat 33 Fiber 13 Carbs 3.9 Protein 23

40. Roasted Cauliflower with Prosciutto, Capers, and Almonds

Preparation Time: 5 Minutes

Cooking Time: 23 minutes

Servings: 4

Ingredients:

- 12 ounces' cauliflower florets (I get precut florets at Trader Joe's)
- 2 tablespoons leftover bacon grease, or olive oil
- Pink Himalayan salt
- Freshly ground black pepper
- 2 ounces sliced prosciutto, torn into small pieces
- 1/4 cup slivered almonds
- 2 tablespoons capers
- 2 tablespoons grated Parmesan cheese

Directions:

1. Preheat the oven to 400F. Line a baking pan with a silicone baking mat or parchment paper.

2. Put the cauliflower florets in the prepared baking pan with the bacon grease, and season with pink Himalayan salt and pepper. Or if you are using olive oil instead, drizzle the cauliflower with olive oil and season with pink Himalayan salt and pepper.

3. Roast the cauliflower for 15 minutes.

4. Stir the cauliflower so all sides are coated with the bacon grease.

5. Distribute the prosciutto pieces in the pan. Then add the slivered almonds and capers. Stir to combine. Sprinkle the Parmesan cheese on top, and roast for 10 minutes more.

6. Divide between two plates, using a slotted spoon so you don't get excess grease in the plates, and serve.

Nutrition: Calories: 576; Total Fat: 48g; Carbs: 1.4g; Fiber: 6g; Protein: 28g

VEGETABLES RECIPES

41. Eggplant Pizza with Tofu

Preparation Time: 15 minutes

Cooking Time: 45 minutes

Servings: 2

Ingredients:

- 2 eggplants, sliced
- 1/3 cup butter, melted
- 2 garlic cloves, minced
- red onion
- 12 oz tofu, chopped
- oz tomato sauce
- Salt and black pepper to taste
- 1/2 tsp. cinnamon powder
- 1 cup Parmesan cheese, shredded
- 1/4 cup dried oregano

Directions:

1. Let the oven heat to 400F. Lay the eggplant slices in a baking sheet and brush with some butter. Bake in the oven until lightly browned, about 20 minutes.

2. Heat the remaining butter in a skillet; sauté garlic and onion until fragrant and soft, about 3 minutes.

3. Stir in the tofu and cook for 3 minutes. Add the tomato sauce, salt and black pepper. Simmer for 10 minutes.

4. Sprinkle with the Parmesan cheese and oregano. Bake for 10 minutes.

Nutrition: Calories: 321 Fat: 11.3g Fiber: 8.4g Carbohydrates: 4.3 g Protein: 10.1g

42. **Brussel Sprouts with Spiced Halloumi**

Preparation Time: 20 minutes

Cooking Time: 30 minutes

Servings: 2

Ingredients:

- 10 oz halloumi cheese, sliced
- tbsp. coconut oil
- 1/2 cup unsweetened coconut, shredded
- 1 tsp. chili powder
- 1/2 tsp. onion powder
- 1/2 pound Brussels sprouts, shredded
- 4 oz butter
- Salt and black pepper to taste
- Lemon wedges for serving

Directions:

1. In a bowl, mix the shredded coconut, chili powder, salt, coconut oil, and onion powder.
2. Then, toss the halloumi slices in the spice mixture.
3. The grill pan must be heated then cook the coated halloumi cheese for 2-3 minutes.
4. Transfer to a plate to keep warm.
5. The half butter must be melted in a pan, add, and sauté the Brussels sprouts until slightly caramelized.

6. Then, season with salt and black pepper.

7. Dish the Brussels sprouts into serving plates with the halloumi cheese and lemon wedges.

8. Melt left butter and drizzle over the Brussels sprouts and halloumi cheese. Serve.

Nutrition: Calories: 276 Fat,: 9.5g Fiber: 9.1g Carbohydrates: 4.1 g Protein: 5.4g

43. Vegetable Patties

Preparation Time: 15 minutes

Cooking Time: 20 minutes

Servings: 4

Ingredients:

- tbsp. olive oil
- 1 onion, chopped
- 1 garlic clove, minced
- 1/2 head cauliflower, grated
- 1 carrot, shredded
- 1tbsp. coconut flour
- 1/2 cup Gruyere cheese, shredded
- 1/2 cup Parmesan cheese, grated
- 3eggs, beaten
- 1/2 tsp. dried rosemary
- Salt and black pepper, to taste

Directions:

1. Cook onion and garlic in warm olive oil over medium heat, until soft, for about 3 minutes.

2. Stir in grated cauliflower and carrot and cook for a minute; allow cooling and set aside.

3. To the cooled vegetables, add the rest of the ingredients, form balls from the mixture, then press each ball to form burger patty.

4. Set oven to 400 F and bake the burgers for 20 minutes.

5. Flip and bake for another 10 minutes or until the top become golden brown.

Nutrition: Calories: 315 Fat: 12.1g Fiber: 8.6g Carbohydrates: 3.3 g Protein: 5.8g

POULTRY RECIPES

44. Rind and Cheese Crusted Chicken

Preparation time: 10 minutes

Cooking time: 10 minutes

Servings: 3

Ingredients:

- 2tablespoons double cream
- 1egg
- 2ounces (57 g) pork rinds, crushed
- 2ounces (57 g) Romano cheese, grated
- Sea salt and ground black pepper, to taste
- 1teaspoon cayenne pepper
- 1teaspoon dried parsley1garlic clove, halved
- ½ pound (227 g) chicken fillets
- 2tablespoons olive oil
- 1large-sized Roma tomato, puréed

Directions:

1. In a mixing bowl, whisk the cream and egg.
2. In another bowl, mix the crushed pork rinds, Romano cheese, salt, black pepper, cayenne pepper, and dried parsley.

3. Rub the garlic halves all over the chicken. Dip the chicken fillets into the egg mixture; then, coat the chicken with breading on all sides.

4. Heat the olive oil in a pan over medium-high heat; add butter. Once hot, cook chicken fillets until no longer pink, 2to 4 minutes on each side.

5. Transfer the prepared chicken fillets to a baking pan that is lightly greased with a nonstick cooking spray. Cover with the puréed tomato. Bake for 2to 3 minutes until everything is thoroughly warmed. Bon appétit!

Nutrition: calories: 360 fats: 23.5g protein: 30.5g carbs: 5.7g net carbs: 3.4g fiber: 1.3g

45. Italian Turkey Meatballs with Leeks

Preparation time: 10 minutes

Cooking time: 20 minutes

Servings: 4

Ingredients:

- 1pound (454 g) ground turkey
- 1tablespoon Italian seasoning blend
- 2cloves garlic, minced
- ½ cup leeks, minced
- 1egg

Directions:

1. Throw all ingredients into a mixing bowl; mix to combine well.

2. Form the mixture into bite-sized balls and arrange them on a parchment-lined baking pan. Spritz the meatballs with cooking spray.

3. Bake in the preheated oven at 400ºF (205ºC) for 18 to 22minutes. Serve with cocktail sticks and enjoy!

Nutrition: calories: 217 fats: 11.1g protein: 24.1g carbs: 3.4g net carbs: 2.8g fiber: 0.6g

46. Chicken Mélange

Preparation time: 15 minutes

Cooking time: 35 minutes

Servings: 3

Ingredients:

- 2ounces (57 g) bacon, diced
- ¾ pound (340 g) whole chicken, boneless and chopped
- ½ medium-sized leek, chopped
- 1teaspoon ginger garlic paste
- 1teaspoon poultry seasoning mix
- Sea salt, to taste
- 1bay leaf
- 1thyme sprig
- 1rosemary sprig
- 1cup chicken broth
- ½ cup cauliflower, chopped into small florets
- 2vine-ripe tomatoes, puréed

Directions:

1. Heat a medium-sized pan over medium-high heat; once hot, fry the bacon until it is crisp or about 3 minutes. Add in the chicken and cook until it is no longer pink; reserve.

2. Then, sauté the leek until tender and fragrant. Stir in the ginger garlic paste, poultry seasoning mix, salt, bay leaf, thyme, and rosemary.

3. Pour in the chicken broth and reduce the heat to medium; let it cook for 15 minutes, stirring periodically.

4. Add in the cauliflower and tomatoes along with the reserved bacon and chicken. Decrease the temperature to simmer and let it cook for a further 15 minutes or until warmed through. Bon appétit!

Nutrition: calories: 353 fats: 14.4g protein: 44.1g carbs: 5.9g net carbs: 3.5g fiber: 2.4g

47. Chicken, Pepper, and Tomato Bake

Preparation time: 10 minutes

Cooking time: 25 minutes

Servings: 3

Ingredients:

- 1tablespoon olive oil
- ¾ pound (340 g) chicken breast fillets, chopped into bite-sized chunks
- 2garlic cloves, sliced
- ¼ teaspoon Korean chili pepper flakes
- ¼ teaspoon Himalayan salt
- ½ teaspoon poultry seasoning mix
- 1bell pepper, deveined and chopped
- 2ripe tomatoes, chopped
- ¼ cup heavy whipping cream
- ¼ cup sour cream

Directions:

1. Brush a casserole dish with olive oil. Add the chicken, garlic, Korean chili pepper flakes, salt, and poultry seasoning mix to the casserole dish.

2. Next, layer the pepper and tomatoes. Whisk the heavy whipping cream and sour cream in a mixing bowl.

3. Top everything with the cream mixture. Bake in the preheated oven at 390ºF (199ºC) for about 25 minutes or until thoroughly heated. Bon appétit!

Nutrition: calories: 411 fats: 20.6g protein: 50.0g carbs: 6.2g net carbs: 4.7g fiber: 1.5g

48. Chicken Quesadilla

Preparation Time: 15 minutes

Cooking Time: 25 minutes

Servings: 4

Ingredients:

- 1tbsp. extra-virgin olive oil
- 1bell pepper, sliced
- 1/2yellow onion, sliced
- 1/2tsp. chili powder
- Kosher salt
- Freshly ground black pepper
- 3 c. shredded Monterey Jack
- 3 c. shredded cheddar
- 4 c. shredded chicken
- 1avocado, thinly sliced
- 1green onion, thinly sliced
- Sour cream, for serving

Directions:

1. Let the oven preheat to 400F.
2. Prepare two baking sheets with a baking mat or parchment paper.
3. Heat oil.

4. Put pepper and onion and season with chili powder, salt, and pepper.

5. Cook until soft, 5 minutes. Transfer to a plate.

6. In a medium bowl, stir together cheeses.

7. Put 11/2cups of cheese mixture onto both prepared baking sheets centers.

8. Spread the cheese evenly in a circle shape, like a flour tortilla.

9. Bake the quesadilla for about 20 minutes.

10. Put onion-pepper mixture, shredded chicken, and avocado slices to one half of each.

11. Let cool slightly.

12. Then use the parchment paper and a little spatula to gently lift.

13. Fold the cheese tortillas empty side over the filling side.

14. Place the quesadilla baking sheet in the oven to heat, 3 to 5 minutes more.

15. Decorate with green onion and sour cream and serve.

Nutrition: Calories: 299 Fat: 12.1g Fiber: 4.1g Carbohydrates: 4.1g Protein: 10.1g

FISH AND SEAFOOD RECIPES

49. Brussel Sprouts with Bacon

Preparation Time: 5 minutes

Cooking Time: 40 minutes

Servings: 6

Ingredients:

- 16 ounces Brussel sprouts
- 1teaspoon salt
- 16 ounces' bacon, pasteurized
- 2/3 teaspoon ground black pepper

Directions:

1. Preheat oven to 400ºF.
2. Slice every sprout in half and then slice bacon lengthwise into small pieces.
3. Take a baking sheet, line it with parchment paper, spread Brussel sprouts halves and bacon on it, and then season with salt and black pepper.
4. Bake for 35–40 minutes until sprouts turn golden-brown, and bacon is crisp.
5. Serve straight away.

Nutrition: Calories: 101 Fat: 5.1g Fiber: 10g Carbohydrates: 1g Protein: 5.5g

50. Grilled Mediterranean Veggies

Preparation Time: 10 minutes

Cooking Time: 15 minutes

Servings: 4

Ingredients:

- 1/4 cup (56 g/2oz) ghee or butter
- 2small (200 g/7.1oz) red, orange, or yellow peppers
- 3 media (600 g/21.2oz) zucchini
- 1medium (500 g/17.6 oz) eggplant
- 1medium (100 g/3.5 oz) red onion

Directions:

1. Set the oven to broil to the highest setting.
2. In a small bowl, mix the melted ghee and crushed garlic.
3. Wash all the vegetables.
4. Halve, deseed, and slice the bell peppers into strips.
5. Slice the zucchini widthwise into 1/4-inch (about 1/2cm) pieces.
6. Wash the eggplant and slice.
7. Quarter each slice into 1/4-inch (about 1/2cm) pieces.
8. Peel and slice the onion into medium wedges and separate the sections using your hands.

9. Place the vegetables in a bowl and add the chopped herbs, ghee with garlic, salt, and black pepper. The vegetables must be spread on a baking sheet, ideally on a roasting rack or net, so that the vegetables don't become soggy from the juices.

10. Put it in the oven and let it cook for about 15 minutes.

11. Be careful not to burn them.

12. When done, the vegetables should be slightly tender but still crisp.

13. Serve with meat dishes or bake with cheese such as feta, mozzarella, or Halloumi.

Nutrition: Calories: 176 Fat: 4.5g Fiber: 9.3g Carbohydrates: 3.1g Protein: 5.2g

51. Bacon and Wild Mushrooms

Preparation Time: 10 minutes

Cooking Time: 10-15 minutes

Servings: 4

Ingredients:

- strips uncured bacon, chopped
- 4 cups sliced wild mushrooms
- 2teaspoons minced garlic
- 2tablespoons chicken stock
- 1tablespoon chopped fresh thyme

Directions:

1. Cook the bacon. In a pot, cook the bacon until it's crispy and cooked through, about 7 minutes.
2. Cook the mushrooms. Add the mushrooms and garlic and sauté until the mushrooms are tender about 7 minutes.
3. Deglaze the pan. Add the chicken stock and stir to scrape up any browned bits in the bottom of the pan.
4. Garnish and serve. Put the mushrooms in a bowl, sprinkle them with the thyme, and serve.

Nutrition: Calories: 175 Fat: 4.9g Fiber: 8.4g Carbohydrates: 2.2g Protein: 1.4g

52. Berries & Spinach Salad

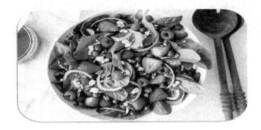

Preparation time: 10 minutes

Cooking time: 0 minutes

Servings: 5

Ingredients:

- Salad
- 8 cups fresh baby spinach
- ¾ cup fresh strawberries, hulled and sliced
- ¾ cup fresh blueberries
- ¼ cup onion, sliced
- ¼ cup almond, sliced
- ¼ cup feta cheese, crumbled
- Dressing
- 1/3 cup olive oil
- 2 tablespoons fresh lemon juice
- ¼ teaspoon liquid stevia

- 1/8 teaspoon garlic powder
- Salt, to taste

Directions:

1. For salad: In a bowl, add the spinach, berries, onion, and almonds, and mix.
2. For dressing: In another small bowl, add all the ingredients and beat until well combined.
3. Place the dressing over salad and gently, toss to coat well.

Nutrition: Calories 190 Net Carbs 6 g Total Fat 17.2 g Saturated Fat 3.3 g Cholesterol 7 mg Sodium 145 mg Total Carbs 8.5 g Fiber 2.5 g Sugar 4.6 g Protein 3.3 g

53. Egg & Avocado Salad

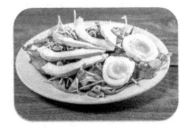

Preparation time: 10 minutes

Cooking time: 0 minutes

Servings: 4

Ingredients:

- **Dressing**
- 3 tablespoons olive oil
- 1 tablespoon fresh lime juice
- Salt and ground black pepper, to taste
- Salad
- 5 cups fresh baby greens
- 4 hard-boiled organic eggs, peeled and sliced
- 2 avocados; peeled, pitted, and sliced
- 2 tablespoons fresh mint leaves

Directions:

1. For dressing: Place oil, lime juice, salt, and black pepper in a small bowl and beat until well combined.

2. Divide the spinach onto serving plates and top each with tuna, egg, cucumber, and tomato.

3. Drizzle with dressing and serve.

Nutrition: Calories 332 Net Carbs 2.5 g Total Fat 31.5 g Saturated Fat 6.4 g Cholesterol 164 mg Sodium 111 mg Total Carbs 8.8 g Fiber 6.3 g Sugar 1.2 g Protein 7.7 g

DESSERT

54. Choco Lava Cake

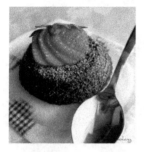

Preparation Time: 15 Minutes

Cooking Time: 45 minutes

Servings: 4

Ingredients:

- ounces of dark chocolate
- 1tablespoon almond flour
- 1/4 cup coconut oil
- 1/4 teaspoon Vanilla extract
- 2eggs
- Cocoa powder for garnish
- 2tablespoons of sweetener

Directions:

1. Preheat the oven to 190C. Grease two molds with coconut oil and sprinkle them with cocoa powder. Melt

chocolate, coconut oil and add vanilla to it. Beat eggs and sweetener together in a different bowl.

2. Slowly add the chocolate mixture with egg mixture and beat until well mixed. Add the almond flour and mix until incorporated. Fill the molds evenly with the mixture. Bake for 10 minutes. Serve immediately.

Nutrition: Calories 126 Fat 9 Fiber 5.46 Carbs 2 Protein 114

55. Coconut Cup Cakes

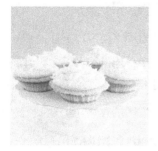

Preparation Time: 15 Minutes

Cooking Time: 45 minutes

Servings: 4

Ingredients:

- Cupcakes:
- 6 tablespoons of coconut flour
- 1/2cup hot water
- 1/2cup unsalted coconut butter
- 1teaspoon vanilla extract
- 1tablespoon flaxseed
- 1teaspoon baking powder
- 4 tablespoons of stevia
- Pinch of salt
- For icing:
- 1cup of raw cashews
- 2tablespoons of Swerve
- 1/2cup whole coconut milk

- 1teaspoon vanilla extract

Directions:

1. Cupcakes:

2. Preheat the oven to 170 C. Grease 6 cupcake molds. Pour the water over the coconut butter and mix well, then add flaxseed, vanilla, stevia, and salt. Leave the flaxseed for few minutes to stow everything. In another bowl, mix baking powder and coconut flour.

3. Add flour mixture and flaxseed mixture slowly and stir until no lumps are left and everything is smooth. Spread them in molds and bake for 20 to 25 minutes until the top is solid and the edges turn golden. Take them out of the oven and wait a few minutes for them to cool

4. Icing

5. Put all ingredients in a blender and blend for about 2-3 minutes until smooth. Add them to cupcakes. Sprinkle with dried coconut if you want

Nutrition: Calories 321 Fat 15 Fiber 5 Carbs 3 Protein 11

CONCLUSION

In the grocery store, the best foods to buy are meats, eggs, non-starchy vegetables, berries and nuts. This does not mean that you need to limit yourself to only these foods. In fact, there are plenty of other keto-friendly options available to you at the store. Just make sure that you read the labels so that you know just how much carbohydrate is in each serving.

These keto-friendly options include:

- Almond flour
- Avocados
- Bacon
- Butter
- Coconut milk
- Full fat cheese (goat, cheddar, mozzarella)
- Healthy oils (olive oil, avocado oil)
- Nuts/seeds (almonds, walnuts, flax seeds)
- Olives and olive oil spreads. (Make sure the spread does not have added sugar.)
- Plain Greek yogurt (with no added sugar). Choose full fat and unsweetened. Plain non-fat Greek yogurt can also be used in recipes to add creaminess.
- Red wine
- Sugar free condiments (mustard, hot sauce, salsa, etc.)

What to eat: Meat (beef/pork/chicken), eggs, non-starchy vegetables, berries and nuts. And you can use unsweetened cocoa powder as a low-carb replacement for chocolate.

What to avoid: Grains (bread, cereal, pasta), sugar and sweeteners (sugar, honey, agave), most fruits and high carb vegetables like potatoes. There's no hard or fast rule here as every person's body is different so some of these may be okay in small amounts.

How To Eat Less & Still Feel Full

One of the most common complaints that people have when starting on a low carb diet is that they are hungry all of the time. They also complain that if they reduce their fat intake, they are not only hungry but feel like they are starving themselves as well.

When you reduce the amount of carbohydrates that you consume, it is natural for your body's metabolism to slow down a bit. Because your metabolism is slowed, you will be able to feel hungry more often than you normally would.

In addition to this, when burning fat for energy, people tend to feel unsatisfied and hungry even after eating a large amount of food. This happens because when food is burned off as energy, there are no nutrients left in the body. This causes people to feel unsatisfied and hungry. Even though they have recently eaten a very large meal, their bodies are still craving nutrients and minerals that are not found in fat alone.